DASH DIET ACTION PLAN

Table of Contents

Introduction

If your purpose is to achieve good wellbeing and to be healthier, then you obviously ended up in the right place! You are about to discover the tool that will benefit your life today. Yeah, this is a diet we're talking about, but not just any diet! We're going to learn about the Diet by Dash!

The Dash diet stands for Hypertension Nutritional Approaches to Stop. This diet reduces your blood pressure and does boost your physical health in no time. Here are few more major health benefits that this incredible diet has brought: This would lower the risk of cancer, your cholesterol will be lowered, this would reduce the risk of diabetes. This would lower the risk of osteoporosis. This would motivate you to reduce more weight. In order to accomplish all these targets, the first thing you have to do is to minimize the ingestion of sodium to no more than 2300 mg per day and to start eating foods that are healthy.

You will consume a lot of veggies, fruits, grains, seeds, natural oils, and nuts during this diet. Low-fat dairy products, cereals, and whole grains, poultry, fish, and seafood Few lean foods, but you have to give up much of the diet of fat and sugar. You can also use frozen ingredients to make dash meals for you, just make sure low-sodium or no-salt-added ones are your choices. The diet for Dash is not a strict one! There are a lot of tasty and perfect ones with the foods you are authorized to consume, you will make meals! So, if you've wanted to start this new life and adopt a dash diet, then you've chosen to follow a dash diet.

The DASH Diet is now attracting popularity for its work for many years, the power to lower blood pressure and the body's vulnerability to wide-ranging Both kinds of ailments. DASH stands for dietary approaches to stop hypertension, an originally developed routine offered to patients seeking to eliminate sodium in their foods; under the DASH Diet, the idea is that a lowered sodium intake contributes to lowered blood pressure, and this is also the ideal routine for those who strive to be safe and stop blood pressure. Except those who were brought on the DASH Diet in the process realized they had lost weight too! Therefore, the DASH Diet was introduced to the community. In the 1990s, when the DASH diet was established, it initially incorporated a staple of carbohydrates and starchy foods. Ultimately, it was changed to the shape that today we see a diet relying on an excess of fresh fruit and vegetables, low-fat meats, and nutritious proteins include seeds, beans, and nuts.

In addition, healthy whole grains like whole-wheat bread are permitted as part of the diet, but in moderation—the empty carbohydrates used in standardized products. For, e.g., white bread and other items are cut out of the diet, seeing how they put on the calories and add to blood pressure. It has been shown by those who adhere closely to the DASH Diet to be one of the most effective ways to reduce lbs. And their bodies all over better.

The DASH Diet is typically split into two stages: Stage One. It lasts two weeks and is supposed to target abdominal fat. Stage Two. Takes in more Food, which was not permitted in the first two weeks and which is the longest-lasting. The stage is said to be the one on which dieters continue for the remainder of their lives. No wonder what the reason for starting the DASH Diet, the advantages of It is not possible to question this regiment, since they lead to a healthy body overall.

What's A Diet For DASH?

DASH is a prescribed diet for those who wish to avoid or treat hypertension — commonly known as high blood pressure — and decrease the risk of heart failure. The focus of the DASH diet is on vegetables, fruit, whole grains, and lean meats. The diet was introduced after research discovered that even in people who adopted a plant-based diet, like vegetarians and vegans, high blood pressure was far less severe.
This is why the DASH diet, while including certain lean protein sources such as fish, chicken, and beans, vegetables, and fruit. The diet consists of low amounts of salt, red meat, added sugar, and fat.
One of the key reasons people with high blood pressure will benefit from this diet, scientists say, is that it decreases the consumption of sodium. The daily DASH diet regimen supports a maximum of 1 tsp (2,300 mg) of sodium each day, which is consistent with other national recommendations. The lower-salt variant suggests no more than 1500 mg (3/4 teaspoon) of sodium a day.

Why DASH Diet

With the vast number of diets available today, it can be hard to detach one that fits with your sort of body and habits. Luckily, there are several those who seem to work for people at a broader level, even though their ambitions are varying significantly. For example, the DASH Diet is a dietary regimen that is initially intended for people with elevated blood pressure or hypertension. Doctors and nutritionists pointed out that their blood pressure had risen. Patients drank sodium, and hence DASH was developed to put its low-sodium diet patients. Even so, the advantage of the DASH Diet is that the patients found that they lost weight.

In addition to lowering their blood pressure, it has now been one of the most common diets since the 1990s has appeared. Among the others, the justification for preferring the DASH Diet is the flexibility it gives for those who prefer it. Made it one of their routines every day. Firstly, there is a choice for the Sodium levels: for those who wish their sodium intake to decline clearly, they may opt for a normal intake dose of 2.300 mg. For the ones who want to exclude from their daily diet a large amount of sodium, the daily intake is limited to 1,500 mg. Which, again, provides Any flexibility. Even the DASH diet is not fully stringent, as some diets are recognized.

A big benefit of this diet is the ability to do so in two stages. The first period lasts about two weeks, and the dieter lasts through this time. Starchy foods and sugars should be avoided as far as possible. This is required to ensure for the first two weeks, the full amount of belly fat is lost. In the 2nd Step, the reintroduction of some good starches into the diet with the mindset that the body still has the enhanced metabolism to cope with them. Dentures start losing weight and are willing to stick to Phase Two as long as In the long run, probably. Another benefit of this diet is that the Step Two diet is so consistent with Eating trends that people still rely on basic shifts, including Whole grains and treats packed with protein are zero. There isn't a lot going on., but a huge advantage once all is said and finished.

Recipes

Breakfast

1 Eggs and Broccoli Casserole

Preparation time: 10 minutes

Cooking time: 4 hours

Servings: 8

Ingredients:

A pinch of black pepper

8 eggs

1 teaspoon garlic, minced

½ yellow onion, chopped

2 bell peppers, chopped

¾ cup low-fat milk

2 teaspoons mustard

1 small broccoli head, florets separated

30 ounces hash browns

Directions:

In a bowl, mix the eggs with the milk, mustard, garlic, hash browns, onion, bell peppers, broccoli and black pepper, stir, pour into your slow cooker, cover and cook on Low for 4 hours.

Divide between plates and serve.

Nutrition: Calories 373, Fat .18.3g, Cholesterol 165mg, Sodium 438mg, Carbohydrate 42.5g, Fiber 4.2g, Sugars 5.1g, Protein 10.3g, Potassium 796mg

2 Blueberries Oatmeal

Preparation time: 10 minutes

Cooking time: 2 hours

Servings: 4

Ingredients:

2 cups non-fat milk

1 cup old fashioned oats

1 cup blueberries

2 teaspoons sugar

½ teaspoon cinnamon powder

½ teaspoon vanilla extract

½ teaspoon almond extract

Directions:

1. In your slow cooker, combine the oats with the milk, berries and the other ingredients, put the lid on and cook on High for 2 hours.

2. Divide the oatmeal into bowls and serve for breakfast.

Nutrition: Calories 231, Fat .2.7g, Cholesterol 2mg, Sodium 65mg, Carbohydrate 40.2g, Fiber 4.8g, Sugars 12.7g, Protein 9.3g, Potassium 391mg

3 Mexican Eggs

Preparation time: 5 minutes

Cooking time: 2 hours

Servings: 8

Ingredients:

12 ounces low-fat cheese, shredded

1 garlic clove, minced

1 cup nonfat sour cream

10 eggs

Olive oil cooking spray

5 ounces canned green chilies, drained

10 ounces tomato sauce, sodium-free

½ teaspoon chili powder

Black pepper to the taste

Directions:

In a bowl, mix the eggs with the cheese, sour cream, chili powder, black pepper, garlic, green chilies and tomato sauce, whisk, pour into your slow cooker after you've greased it with cooking oil, cover and cook on Low for 2 hours.

Divide between plates and serve.

Nutrition: Calories 395, Fat .27.5g, Cholesterol 262mg, Sodium 700mg, Carbohydrate 18.8g, Fiber 5.8g, Sugars 10.6g, Protein 20.9g, Potassium 610mg

4 Cherry Tomatoes Bowls

Preparation time: 10 minutes

Cooking time: 1 hour

Servings: 4

Ingredients:

1 cup pomegranate seeds

½ cup low-sodium veggie stock

½ pound cherry tomatoes, halved

1 teaspoon turmeric powder

1 tablespoon basil, chopped

A pinch of cayenne pepper

Directions:

1. In your slow cooker, combine the tomatoes with the pomegranate seeds and the other ingredients, put the lid on and cook on High for 1 hour.

2. Divide into bowls and serve.

Nutrition: Calories 57, Fat .0.2g, Cholesterol 0mg, Sodium 21mg, Carbohydrate 13.2g, Fiber 1.3g, Sugars 6.8g, Protein 1g, Potassium 151mg

5 Coconut Sugar Oatmeal

Preparation time: 5 minutes

Cooking time: 10 hours

Servings: 4

Ingredients:

2 teaspoons low-fat butter

4 apples, peeled, cored and chopped

1 and ½ tablespoon cinnamon powder

1 cup coconut sugar

2 cups old-fashioned oats

4 cups coconut water

Directions:

Grease your slow cooker with the butter, add apples, coconut sugar, cinnamon, oats and water, cover and cook on Low for 10 hours.

Stir the oatmeal, divide into bowls and serve.

Nutrition: Calories 421, Fat .30g, Cholesterol 0mg, Sodium 40mg, Carbohydrate 43g, Fiber 8.2g, Sugars 27.4g, Protein 4.1g, Potassium 554mg

6 Sweet Chia Bowls

Preparation time: 10 minutes

Cooking time: 2 hours

Servings: 4

Ingredients:

2 cups non-fat milk

1 cup brown rice

2 bananas, peeled and sliced

1 tablespoon maple syrup

2 tablespoons chia seeds

1 teaspoon sugar

1 teaspoon vanilla extract

1 teaspoon cinnamon powder

Directions:

1. In your slow cooker, combine the milk with the bananas, maple syrup and the other ingredients, put the lid on and cook on High for 2 hours.

2. Divide the mix into bowls and serve for breakfast.

Nutrition: Calories 321, Fat .3.5g, Cholesterol 3mg, Sodium 69mg, Carbohydrate 63.4g, Fiber 5.4g, Sugars 17.3g, Protein 9.3g, Potassium 577mg

7 Maple Quinoa with Cut Oats

Preparation time: 10 minutes

Cooking time: 7 hours

Servings: 6

Ingredients:

2 tablespoons stevia

2 tablespoons maple syrup

½ cup quinoa

½ teaspoon vanilla extract

1 and ½ cups steel cut oats

4 cups water

Directions:

In your slow cooker, mix the oats with the quinoa, water, stevia, maple syrup and vanilla, cover and cook on Low for 7 hours.

Stir the oatmeal, divide it into bowls and serve.

Nutrition: Calories 148, Fat 2.2g, Cholesterol 0mg, Sodium 7mg, Carbohydrate 32.4g, Fiber 3.1g, Sugars 4.2g, Protein 4.7g, Potassium 170mg

---

Soup

8 Ginger Zucchini Avocado Soup

Preparation time: 15 minutes

Cooking time: 25 minutes

Servings: 3

Ingredients:

1 red bell pepper, chopped

1 big avocado

1 teaspoon ginger, grated

Pepper as needed

2 tablespoons avocado oil

4 scallions, chopped

1 tablespoon lemon juice

29 ounces vegetable stock

1 garlic clove, minced

2 zucchinis, chopped

1 cup of water

Directions:

Take a pan and place over medium heat, add onion and fry for 3 minutes. Stir in ginger, garlic and cook for 1 minute. Mix in seasoning, zucchini stock, water, and boil for 10 minutes. Remove soup from fire and let it sit; blend in avocado and blend using an immersion blender. Heat over low heat for a while. Adjust your seasoning and add lemon juice, bell pepper. Serve and enjoy!

Nutrition: Calories: 155 Fat: 11g Carbohydrates: 10g Protein: 7g Sodium: 345 mg

9   Greek Lemon and Chicken Soup

Preparation time: 15 minutes

Cooking time: 30 minutes

Servings: 4

Ingredients:

2 cups cooked chicken, chopped

2 medium carrots, chopped

½ cup onion, chopped

¼ cup lemon juice

1 clove garlic, minced

1 can cream of chicken soup, fat-free and low sodium

2 cans of chicken broth, fat-free

¼ teaspoon ground black pepper

2/3 cup long-grain rice

2 tablespoons parsley, snipped

Directions:

Put all of the listed fixings in a pot (except rice and parsley). Season with sunflower seeds and pepper. Bring the mix to a boil over medium-high heat. Stir in rice and set heat to medium.

Simmer within 20 minutes until rice is tender. Garnish parsley and enjoy!

Nutrition: Calories: 582 Fat: 33g Carbohydrates: 35g Protein: 32g Sodium: 210 mg

10   Garlic and Pumpkin Soup

Preparation time: 15 minutes

Cooking time: 5 hours

Servings: 4

Ingredients:

1-pound pumpkin chunks

1 onion, diced

2 cups vegetable stock

1 2/3 cups coconut cream

½ stick almond butter

1 teaspoon garlic, crushed

1 teaspoon ginger, crushed

Pepper to taste

Directions:

Add all the fixing into your Slow Cooker. Cook for 4-6 hours on high. Puree the soup by using your immersion blender. Serve and enjoy!

Nutrition: Calories: 235 Fat: 21g Carbohydrates: 11g Protein: 2g Sodium: 395 mg

11   Golden Mushroom Soup

Preparation time: 15 minutes

Cooking time: 8 hours

Servings: 6

Ingredients:

1 onion, finely chopped

1 carrot, peeled and finely chopped

1 fennel bulb, finely chopped

1-pound fresh mushrooms, quartered

8 cups Vegetable Broth, Poultry Broth, or store-bought

¼ cup dry sherry

1 teaspoon dried thyme

1 teaspoon garlic powder

½ teaspoon of sea salt

1/8 teaspoon freshly ground black pepper

Directions:

In your slow cooker, combine all the ingredients, mixing to combine. Cover and set on low. Cook for 8 hours.

Nutrition: Calories: 71 Fat: 0g Carbohydrates: 15g Fiber: 3g Protein: 3g Sodium: 650 mg

---

Meat

12   Pork Patties

Preparation time: 10 minutes

Cooking time: 35 minutes

Servings: 6

Ingredients:

½ cup coconut flour

2 tablespoons olive oil

2 egg, whisked

Black pepper to the taste

1 and ½ pounds pork, ground

10 ounces low sodium veggie stock

¼ cup tomato sauce, no-salt-added

½ teaspoon mustard powder

Directions:

Put the flour in a bowl and the egg in another one.

Mix the pork with black pepper and a pinch of paprika, shape medium patties out of this mix, dip them in the egg and then dredge in flour.

Heat up a pan with the oil over medium-high heat, add the patties and cook them for 5 minutes on each side.

In a bowl, combine the stock with tomato sauce and mustard powder and whisk.

Add this over the patties, cook for 10 minutes over medium heat, divide everything between plates and serve.

Enjoy!

Nutrition: calories 332, fat 18, fiber 4, carbs 11, protein 25

13 Pork Roast with Mushrooms

Preparation time: 10 minutes

Cooking time: 1 hour and 20 minutes

Servings: 4

Ingredients:

3 and ½ pounds pork roast

4 ounces mushrooms, sliced

12 ounces low-sodium beef stock

1 teaspoon Italian seasoning

Directions:

In a roasting pan, combine the roast with mushrooms, stock and Italian seasoning, toss, introduce in the oven and bake at 350 degrees F for 1 hour and 20 minutes.

Slice the roast, divide it and the mushroom mix between plates and serve.

Enjoy!

Nutrition: calories 310, fat 16, fiber 2, carbs 10, protein 22

14   Pork Meatloaf

Preparation time: 10 minutes

Cooking time: 50 minutes

Servings: 6

Ingredients:

1 cup white mushrooms, chopped

3 pounds pork, ground

2 tablespoons parsley, chopped

2 garlic cloves, minced

½ cup yellow onion, chopped

¼ cup red bell pepper, chopped

½ cup almond flour

1/3 cup low-fat parmesan, grated

3 eggs

Black pepper to the taste

1 teaspoon balsamic vinegar

Directions:

In a bowl, mix the pork with the black pepper, bell pepper, mushrooms, garlic, onion, parsley, almond flour, parmesan, vinegar and eggs, stir very well, transfer this into a loaf pan and bake in the oven at 375 degrees F for 50 minutes.

Leave meatloaf to cool down, slice and serve it.

Enjoy!

Nutrition: calories 274, fat 14, fiber 3, carbs 8, protein 24

15   Garlic Meatballs Salad

Preparation time: 10 minutes

Cooking time: 15 minutes

Servings: 6

Ingredients:

17 ounces pork ground

1 yellow onion, grated

1 egg, whisked

¼ cup parsley, chopped

Black pepper to the taste

2 garlic cloves, minced

¼ cup mint, chopped

2 and ½ teaspoons oregano, dried

¼ cup olive oil

7 ounces cherry tomatoes, halved

1 cucumber, thinly sliced

1 cup baby spinach

1 and ½ tablespoons lemon juice

A drizzle of avocado oil

Directions:

In a bowl, combine the pork with the onion, egg, parsley, black pepper, mint, garlic and oregano, stir well and shape medium meatballs out of this mix.

Heat up a pan with the olive oil over medium-high heat, add the meatballs and cook them for 5 minutes on each side.

In a salad bowl, combine the meatballs with the tomatoes, cucumber, spinach, lemon juice and avocado oil, toss and serve.

Enjoy!

Nutrition: calories 220, fat 4, fiber 6, carbs 8, protein 12

16   Meatballs And Sauce

Preparation time: 10 minutes

Cooking time: 32 minutes

Servings: 6

Ingredients:

2 pounds pork, ground

Black pepper to the taste

½ teaspoon garlic powder

1 tablespoon coconut aminos

¼ cup low sodium veggie

¾ cup almond flour

1 tablespoon parsley, chopped

For the sauce:

1 cup yellow onion, chopped

2 cups mushrooms, sliced

2 tablespoons olive oil

1 teaspoon coconut aminos

½ cup coconut cream

Black pepper to the taste

Directions:

In a bowl, mix the pork with black pepper, garlic powder, 1 tablespoons coconut aminos, stock, almond flour and parsley, stir well, shape medium meatballs out of this mix, arrange them on a baking sheet, introduce in the oven at 375 degrees F and bake for 20 minutes.

Meanwhile, heat up a pan with the oil over medium heat, add mushrooms, stir and cook for 4 minutes.

Add onions, 1 teaspoon coconut aminos, cream and black pepper, stir and cook for 5 minutes more.

Add the meatballs, toss gently, cook for 1-2 minutes more, divide everything into bowls and serve.

Enjoy!

Nutrition: calories 435, fat 23, fiber 4, carbs 6, protein 32

Seafood

17   Generous Stuffed Salmon Avocado

Preparation time: 10 minutes

Cooking Time: 30 minutes

Serving: 2

Ingredients:

1 ripe organic avocado

2 ounces wild caught smoked salmon

1 ounce cashew cheese

2 tablespoons extra virgin olive oil

Sunflower seeds as needed

Directions:

Cut avocado in half and deseed.

Add the rest of the ingredients to a food processor and process until coarsely chopped.

Place mixture into avocado.

Serve and enjoy!

Nutrition:

Calories: 525

Fat: 48g

Carbohydrates: 4g

Protein: 19g

18   Spanish Mussels

Preparation time: 10 minutes

Cooking Time: 23 minutes

Serving: 4

Ingredients:

3 tablespoons olive oil

2 pounds mussels, scrubbed

Pepper to taste

3 cups canned tomatoes, crushed

1 shallot, chopped

2 garlic cloves, minced

2 cups low sodium vegetable stock

1/3 cup cilantro, chopped

Directions:

Take a pan and place it over medium-high heat, add shallot and stir-cook for 3 minutes.

Add garlic, stock, tomatoes, pepper, stir and reduce heat, simmer for 10 minutes.

Add mussels, cilantro, and toss.

Cover and cook for 10 minutes more.

Serve and enjoy!

Nutrition:

Calories: 210

Fat: 2g

Carbohydrates: 5g

Protein: 8g

19   Tilapia Broccoli Platter

Preparation time: 4 minutes

Cooking Time: 14 minutes

Serving: 2

Ingredients:

6 ounce tilapia, frozen

1 tablespoon almond butter

1 tablespoon garlic, minced

1 teaspoon lemon pepper seasoning

1 cup broccoli florets, fresh

Directions:

Preheat your oven to 350 degrees F.

Add fish in aluminum foil packets.

Arrange broccoli around fish.

Sprinkle lemon pepper on top.

Close the packets and seal.

Bake for 14 minutes.

Take a bowl and add garlic and almond butter, mix well and keep the mixture on the side.

Remove the packet from oven and transfer to platter.

Place almond butter on top of the fish and broccoli, serve and enjoy!

Nutrition:

Calories: 362

Fat: 25g

Carbohydrates: 2g

Protein: 29g

20 Salmon with Peas and Parsley Dressing

Preparation time: 15 minutes

Cooking Time: 15 minutes

Serving: 4

Ingredients:

16 ounces salmon fillets, boneless and skin-on

1 tablespoon parsley, chopped

10 ounces peas

9 ounces vegetable stock, low sodium

2 cups water

½ teaspoon oregano, dried

½ teaspoon sweet paprika

2 garlic cloves, minced

A pinch of black pepper

Directions:

Add garlic, parsley, paprika, oregano and stock to a food processor and blend.

Add water to your Instant Pot.

Add steam basket.

Add fish fillets inside the steamer basket.

Season with pepper.

Lock the lid and cook on HIGH pressure for 10 minutes.

Release the pressure naturally over 10 minutes.

Divide the fish amongst plates.

Add peas to the steamer basket and lock the lid again, cook on HIGH pressure for 5 minutes.

Quick release the pressure.

Divide the peas next to your fillets and serve with the parsley dressing drizzled on top

Enjoy!

Nutrition:

Calories: 315

Fat: 5g

Carbohydrates: 14g

Protein: 16g

Vegetarian and Vegan

21   Aromatic Whole Grain Spaghetti

Preparation Time: 5 minutes

Cooking Time: 10 minutes

Servings: 2

Ingredients:

1 teaspoon dried basil

¼ cup of soy milk

6 oz whole-grain spaghetti

2 cups of water

1 teaspoon ground nutmeg

Bring the water to boil, add spaghetti and cook them for 8-10 minutes.

Meanwhile, bring the soy milk to boil.

Drain the cooked spaghetti and mix them up with soy milk, ground nutmeg, and dried basil.

Stir the meal well.

Directions:

Nutrition:

Calories 128

Protein 5.6g

Carbohydrates 25g

Fat 1.4g

Fiber 4.3g

Cholesterol 0mg

Sodium 25mg

Potassium 81mg

22   Chunky Tomatoes

Preparation Time: 5 minutes

Cooking Time: 15 minutes

Servings: 3

Ingredients:

2 cups plum tomatoes, roughly chopped

½ cup onion, diced

½ teaspoon garlic, diced

1 teaspoon Italian seasonings

1 teaspoon canola oil

1 chili pepper, chopped

Directions:

Heat up canola oil in the saucepan.

Add chili pepper and onion. Cook the vegetables for 5 minutes. Stir them from time to time.

After this, add tomatoes, garlic, and Italian seasonings.

Close the lid and sauté the meal for 10 minutes.

Nutrition:

Calories 550

Protein 1.7g

Carbohydrates 8.4g

Fat 2.3g

Fiber 1.8g

Cholesterol 1mg

Sodium 17mg

Potassium 279mg

23   Baked Falafel

Preparation Time: 10 minutes

Cooking Time: 25 minutes

Servings: 6

Ingredients:

2 cups chickpeas, cooked

1 yellow onion, diced

3 tablespoons olive oil

1 cup fresh parsley, chopped

1 teaspoon ground cumin

½ teaspoon coriander

2 garlic cloves, diced

Directions:

Put all ingredients in the food processor and blend until smooth.

Preheat the oven to 375F.

Then line the baking tray with the baking paper.

Make the balls from the chickpeas mixture and press them gently in the shape of the falafel.

Put the falafel in the tray and bake in the oven for 25 minutes.

Nutrition:

Calories 316

Protein 13.5g

Carbohydrates 43.3g

Fat 11.2g

Fiber 12.4g

Cholesterol 0mg

Sodium 23mg

Potassium 676mg

24   Paella

Preparation Time: 10 minutes

Cooking Time: 25 minutes

Servings: 6

Ingredients:

1 teaspoon dried saffron

1 cup short-grain rice

1 tablespoon olive oil

2 cups of water

1 teaspoon chili flakes

6 oz artichoke hearts, chopped

½ cup green peas

1 onion, sliced

1 cup bell pepper, sliced

Directions:

Pour water in the saucepan. Add rice and cook it for 15 minutes.

Meanwhile, heat up olive oil in the skillet.

Add dried saffron, chili flakes, onion, and bell pepper.

Roast the vegetables for 5 minutes.

Add them to the cooked rice.

Then add artichoke hearts and green peas. Stir the paella well and cook it for 10 minutes over the low heat.

Nutrition:

Calories 170

Protein 4.2g

Carbohydrates 32.7g

Fat 2.7g

Fiber 3.2g

Cholesterol 0mg

Sodium 33mg

Potassium 237mg

25 Mushroom Cakes

Preparation Time: 15 minutes

Cooking Time: 10 minutes

Servings: 4

Ingredients:

2 cups mushrooms, chopped

3 garlic cloves, chopped

1 tablespoon dried dill

1 egg, beaten

¼ cup of rice, cooked

1 tablespoon sesame oil

1 teaspoon chili powder

Directions:

Grind the mushrooms in the food processor.

Add garlic, dill, egg, rice, and chili powder.

Blend the mixture for 10 seconds.

After this, heat up sesame oil for 1 minute.

Make the medium size mushroom cakes and put in the hot sesame oil.

Cook the mushroom cakes for 5 minutes per side on the medium heat.

Nutrition:

Calories 103

Protein 3.7g

Carbohydrates 12g

Fat 4.8g

Fiber 0.9g

Cholesterol 41mg

Sodium 27mg

Potassium 187mg

Side Dishes, Salads & Appetizers

26 Unique Eggplant Salad

Preparation time: 10 minutes

Cooking Time: 30 minutes

Serving: 3

Ingredients:

2 eggplants, peeled and sliced

2 garlic cloves

2 green bell pepper, sliced, seeds removed

½ cup fresh parsley

½ cup mayonnaise, low fat, low sodium

Sunflower seeds and black pepper

Directions:

Preheat your oven to 480 degrees F.

Take a baking pan and add eggplant, bell peppers and season with black [MOU15] [F16]pepper to it.

Bake for about 30 minutes.

Flip the vegetables after 20 minutes.

Then, take a bowl, add baked vegetables and all the remaining ingredients.

Mix well.

Serve and enjoy!

Nutrition:

Calories: 196

Fat: 108.g

Carbohydrates: 13.4g

Protein: 14.6g

27 Zucchini Pesto Salad

Preparation time: 10 minutes

Cooking Time: 10 minutes

Serving: 4

Ingredients:

2 cups spiral pasta

2 zucchini, sliced and halved

4 tomatoes, cut

1 cup white mushrooms, cut

1 small red onion, chopped

2 tablespoons fresh basil leaves, chopped

2 tablespoons sunflower oil

1 tablespoon lemon juice

Pepper and sunflower seeds to taste

Directions:

Cook the pasta according to the package instructions, drain and rinse under cold water.

Take a large bowl and add zucchini, tomatoes, mushrooms, onion, and pasta.

Mix well,

In a food processor, add oil, lemon juice, basil, blue cheese, black, and process well.

Pour the mixture over the salad and toss well.

Serve and enjoy!

Nutrition:

Calories: 301

Fat: 25g

Net Carbohydrates: 7g

Protein: 10g

28   Wholesome Potato and Tuna Salad

Preparation time: 10 minutes

Cooking Time: Nil

Serving: 4

Ingredients:

1 pound baby potatoes, scrubbed, boiled

1 cup tuna chunks, drained

1 cup cherry tomatoes, halved

1 cup medium onion, thinly sliced

8 pitted black olives

2 medium hard-boiled eggs, sliced

1 head Romaine lettuce

¼ cup olive oil

2 tablespoons lemon juice

1 tablespoon Dijon mustard

1 teaspoon dill weed, chopped

Pepper as needed

Directions:

Take a small glass bowl and mix in your olive oil, lemon juice, Dijon mustard and dill.

Season the mix with pepper and salt.

Add in the tuna, baby potatoes, cherry tomatoes, red onion, green beans, black olives and toss everything nicely.

Arrange your lettuce leaves on a beautiful serving dish to make the base of your salad.

Top them with your salad mixture and place the egg slices.

Drizzle with the previously prepared Salad Dressing.

Serve hot

Nutrition:

Calories: 406

Fat: 22g

Carbohydrates: 28g

Protein: 26g

29   Baby Spinach Salad

Preparation time: 10 minutes

Cooking Time: Nil

Serving: 2

Ingredients:

1 bag baby spinach, washed and dried

1 red bell pepper, cut in slices

1 cup cherry tomatoes, cut in halves

1 small red onion, finely chopped

1 cup black olives, pitted

For dressing:

1 teaspoon dried oregano

1 large garlic clove

3 tablespoons red wine vinegar

4 tablespoons olive oil

Sunflower seeds and pepper to taste

Directions:

Prepare the dressing by blending in garlic, olive oil, vinegar in a food processor.

Take a large salad bowl and add spinach leaves, toss well with the dressing.

Add remaining ingredients and toss again, season with sunflower seeds and pepper and enjoy!

Nutrition:

Calories: 126

Fat: 10g

Carbohydrates: 10g

Protein: 2g

Preparation time: 10 minutes

Cooking Time: 2 hours

Serving: 6

Ingredients:

2 ounces prosciutto, cut into strips

1 teaspoon olive oil

2 cups corn

1/2 cup salt-free tomato sauce

1 teaspoon garlic, minced

1 green bell pepper, chopped

Directions:

Grease your Slow Cooker with oil.

Add corn, prosciutto, garlic, tomato sauce, bell pepper to your Slow Cooker.

Stir and place lid.

Cook on HIGH for 2 hours.

Divide between serving platters and enjoy!

Nutrition:

Calories: 109

Fat: 2g

Carbohydrates: 10g

Protein: 5g

31   Arabic Fattoush Salad

Preparation time: 15 minutes

Cooking Time: 2-3 minutes

Serving: 4

Ingredients:

1 whole wheat pita bread

1 large English cucumber, diced

2 cup grape tomatoes, halved

½ medium red onion, finely diced

¾ cup fresh parsley, chopped

¾ cup mint leaves, chopped

1 clove garlic, minced

¼ cup fat free feta cheese, crumbled

1 tablespoon olive oil

1 teaspoon ground sumac

Juice from ½ a lemon

Salt and pepper as needed

Directions:

Mist pita bread with cooking spray.

Season with salt.

Toast until the breads are crispy.

Take a large bowl and add the remaining ingredients and mix (except feta).

Top the mix with diced toasted pita and feta.

Serve and enjoy!

Nutrition:

Calories: 86

Fat: 3g

Carbohydrates: 9g

Protein: 9g

32   Heart Warming Cauliflower Salad

Preparation time: 8 minutes

Cooking Time: Nil

Serving: 3

Ingredients:

1 head cauliflower, broken into florets

1 small onion, chopped

1/8 cup extra virgin olive oil

¼ cup apple cider vinegar

½ teaspoon of sea salt

½ teaspoon of black pepper

¼ cup dried cranberries

¼ cup pumpkin seeds

Directions:

Wash the cauliflower and break it up into small florets.

Transfer to a bowl.

Whisk oil, vinegar, salt and pepper in another bowl.

Add pumpkin seeds, cranberries to the bowl with dressing.

Mix well and pour the dressing over the cauliflower.

Add onions and toss.

Chill and serve.

Enjoy!

Nutrition:

Calories: 163

Fat: 11g

Carbohydrates: 16g

Protein: 3g

33   Great Greek Sardine Salad

Preparation time: 10 minutes

Cooking Time: 10 minutes

Serving: 2

Ingredients:

2 tablespoons extra virgin olive oil

1 garlic clove, minced

2 teaspoons dried oregano

½ teaspoon freshly ground pepper

3 medium tomatoes, cut into large sized chunks

1 can (15 ounces) rinsed chickpeas

1/3 cup feta cheese, crumbled

¼ cup red onion, sliced

2 tablespoons Kalamata olives, sliced

2 cans 4 ounce drained sardines, with bones and packed in either oil or water

Directions:

Take a large bowl and whisk in lemon juice, oregano, garlic, oil, pepper and mix well.

Add tomatoes, chickpeas, cucumber, olives, feta and mix.

Divide the salad amongst serving platter and top with sardines.

Enjoy!

Nutrition:

Calories: 347

Fat: 18g

Carbohydrates: 29g

Protein: 17g

34   Shrimp and Egg Medley

Preparation time: 15 minutes

Cooking Time: Nil

Serving: 4

Ingredients:

4 hard boiled eggs, peeled and chopped

1 pound cooked shrimp, peeled and deveined, chopped

1 sprig fresh dill, chopped

¼ cup mayonnaise

1 teaspoon Dijon mustard

4 fresh lettuce leaves

Directions:

Take a large serving bowl and add the listed ingredients (except lettuce).

Stir well.

Serve over bed of lettuce leaves.

Enjoy!

Nutrition:

Calories: 292

Fat: 17g

Carbohydrates: 1.6g

Protein: 30g

Dessert and Snacks

35   Yummy Espresso Fat Bombs

Preparation time: 20 minutes

Cooking time: nil

Freeze Time: 4 hours

Servings: 24

Ingredients:

5 tablespoons butter, tender

3 ounces cream cheese, soft

2 ounces espresso

4 tablespoons coconut oil

2 tablespoons coconut whipping cream

2 tablespoons stevia

Directions:

Prepare your double boiler and melt all ingredients (except stevia) for 3-4 minutes and mix.

Add sweetener and mix using hand mixer.

Spoon mixture into silicone muffin molds and freeze for 4 hours.

Remove fat bombs and enjoy!

Nutrition: Total Carbs: 1.3g Fiber: 0.2g Protein: 0.3g Fat: 7g

36   Crispy Coconut Bombs

Preparation time: 10 minutes

Cooking time: 0 minutes

Freeze Time: 1-2 hours

Servings: 6

Ingredients:

14 ½ ounces coconut milk

¾ cup coconut oil

1 cup unsweetened coconut flakes

20 drops stevia

Directions:

Microwave your coconut oil for 20 seconds in microwave.

Mix in coconut milk and stevia in the hot oil.

Stir in coconut flakes and pour the mixture into molds.

Let it chill for 60 minutes in fridge.

Serve and enjoy!

Nutrition: Total Carbs: 2g Fiber: 0.5g Protein: 1g Fat: 13g

Calories: 123 Net Carbs: 1g

37   Pumpkin Pie Fat Bombs

Preparation time: 35 minutes

Cooking time: 5 minutes

Freeze Time: 3 hours

Servings: 12

Ingredients:

2 tablespoons coconut oil

1/3 cup pumpkin puree

1/3 cup almond oil

¼ cup almond oil

3 ounces sugar-free dark chocolate

1 ½ teaspoons pumpkin pie spice mix

Stevia to taste

Directions:

Melt almond oil and dark chocolate over a double boiler.

Take this mixture and layer the bottom of 12 muffin cups.

Freeze until the crust has set.

Meanwhile, take a saucepan and combine the rest of the ingredients.

Put the saucepan on low heat.

Heat until softened and mix well.

Pour this over the initial chocolate mixture.

Let it chill for at least 1 hour.

Nutrition: Total Carbs: 3g Fiber: 1g Protein: 3g Fat: 13g

Calories: 124

38   Sensational Lemonade Fat Bomb

Preparation time: 2 hours

Cooking time: Nil

Servings: 2

Ingredients:

½ lemon

4 ounces cream cheese

2 ounces almond butter

Salt to taste

2 teaspoons natural sweetener

Directions:

Take a fine grater and zest lemon.

Squeeze lemon juice into bowl with zest.

Add butter, cream cheese in a bowl and add zest, juice, salt, sweetener.

Mix well using a hand mixer until smooth.

Spoon mixture into molds and let them freeze for 2 hours.

Serve and enjoy!

Nutrition: Calories: 404 Fat: 43g Carbohydrates: 4g Protein: 4g

39   Sweet Almond and Coconut Fat Bombs

Preparation time: 10 minutes

Cooking time: 0 minutes

Freeze Time: 20 minutes

Servings: 6

Ingredients:

¼ cup melted coconut oil

9 ½ tablespoons almond butter

90 drops liquid stevia

3 tablespoons cocoa

9 tablespoons melted butter, salted

Directions:

Take a bowl and add all of the listed ingredients.

Mix them well.

Pour scant 2 tablespoons of the mixture into as many muffin molds as you like.

Chill for 20 minutes and pop them out.

Serve and enjoy!

Nutrition: Total Carbs: 2g Fiber: 0g Protein: 2.53g Fat: 14g

40   Almond and Tomato Balls

Preparation time: 10 minutes

Cooking time: 0 minutes

Freeze Time: 20 minutes

Servings: 6

Ingredients:

1/3 cup pistachios, de-shelled

10 ounces cream cheese

1/3 cup sun dried tomatoes, diced

Directions:

Chop pistachios into small pieces.

Add cream cheese, tomatoes in a bowl and mix well.

Chill for 15-20 minutes and turn into balls.

Roll into pistachios.

Serve and enjoy!

Nutrition: Carb: 183 Fat: 18g Carb: 5g Protein: 5g

41   Avocado Tuna Bites

Preparation time: 10 minutes

Cooking time: nil

Servings: 4

Ingredients:

1/3 cup coconut oil

1 avocado, cut into cubes

10 ounces canned tuna, drained

¼ cup parmesan cheese, grated

¼ teaspoon garlic powder

1/4 teaspoon onion powder

1/3 cup almond flour

¼ teaspoon pepper

¼ cup low fat mayonnaise

Pepper as needed

Directions:

Take a bowl and add tuna, mayo, flour, parmesan, spices and mix well.

Fold in avocado and make 12 balls out of the mixture.

Melt coconut oil in pan and cook over medium heat, until all sides are golden.

Serve and enjoy!

Nutrition: Calories: 185 Fat: 18g Carbohydrates: 1g Protein: 5g

42   Mediterranean Pop Corn Bites

Preparation time: 5 minutes + 20 minutes chill time

Cooking time: 2-3 minutes

Servings: 4

Ingredients:

3 cups Medjool dates, chopped

12 ounces brewed coffee

1 cup pecan, chopped

½ cup coconut, shredded

½ cup cocoa powder

Directions:

Soak dates in warm coffee for 5 minutes.

Remove dates from coffee and mash them, making a fine smooth mixture.

Stir in remaining ingredients (except cocoa powder) and form small balls out of the mixture.

Coat with cocoa powder, serve and enjoy!

Nutrition: Calories: 265 Fat: 12g Carbohydrates: 43g Protein 3g

43   Tasty Cucumber Bites

Preparation time: 5 minutes

Cooking time: nil

Servings: 4

Ingredients:

1 (8 ounce) cream cheese container, low fat

1 tablespoon bell pepper, diced

1 tablespoon shallots, diced

1 tablespoon parsley, chopped

2 cucumbers

Pepper to taste

Directions:

Take a bowl and add cream cheese, onion, pepper, parsley.

Peel cucumbers and cut in half.

Remove seeds and stuff with cheese mix.

Cut into bite sized portions and enjoy!

Nutrition: Calories: 85 Fat: 4g Carbohydrates: 2g Protein: 3g

44   Juicy Simple Lemon Fat Bombs

Preparation time: 10 minutes

Cooking time: /

Freeze Time: 2 hours

Servings: 3

Ingredients:

1 whole lemon

4 ounces cream cheese

2 ounces butter

2 teaspoons natural sweetener

Directions:

Take a fine grater and zest your lemon.

Squeeze lemon juice into a bowl alongside the zest.

Add butter, cream cheese to a bowl and add zest, salt, sweetener and juice.

Stir well using a hand mixer until smooth.

Spoon mix into molds and freeze for 2 hours.

Serve and enjoy!

Nutrition: Total Carbs: 4g Fiber: 1g Protein: 4g Fat: 43g Calories: 404

45   Chocolate Coconut Bombs

Preparation time: 20 minutes

Cooking time: None

Freeze Time:1 hour

Servings: 12

Ingredients:

½ cup dark cocoa powder

½tablespoon vanilla extract

5 drops stevia

1 cup coconut oil, solid

1tablespoon peppermint extract

Directions:

Take a high-speed food processor and add all the ingredients. Blend until combined.

Take a teaspoon and drop a spoonful onto parchment paper.

Refrigerate until solidified and keep refrigerated.

Nutrition: Total Carbs: 0g Fiber: 0g Protein: 0g Fat: 14g

Calories: 126

46   Terrific Jalapeno Bacon Bombs

Preparation time: 15 minutes

Cooking time: 10 minutes

Servings: 2

Ingredients:

12 large jalapeno peppers

16 bacon strips

6 ounces full fat cream cheese

2 teaspoon garlic powder

1 teaspoon chili powder

Directions:

Preheat your oven to 350 degrees F.

Place a wire rack over a roasting pan and keep it on the side.

Make a slit lengthways across jalapeno pepper and scrape out the seeds, discard them.

Place a nonstick skillet over high heat and add half of your bacon strips, cook until crispy.

Drain them.

Chop the cooked bacon strips and transfer to large bowl.

Add cream cheese and mix.

Season the cream cheese and bacon mix with garlic and chili powder.

Mix well.

Stuff the mix into the jalapeno peppers with and wrap a raw bacon strip all around.

Arrange the stuffed wrapped jalapeno on prepared wire rack.

Roast for 10 minutes.

Transfer to cooling rack and serve!

Nutrition: Calories: 209 Fat: 9g Net Carbohydrates: 15g Protein: 9g

47   Yummy Espresso Fat Bombs

Preparation time: 20 minutes

Cooking time: nil

Freeze Time: 4 hours

Servings: 24

Ingredients:

5 tablespoons butter, tender

3 ounces cream cheese, soft

2 ounces espresso

4 tablespoons coconut oil

2 tablespoons coconut whipping cream

2 tablespoons stevia

Directions:

Prepare your double boiler and melt all ingredients (except stevia) for 3-4 minutes and mix.

Add sweetener and mix using hand mixer.

Spoon mixture into silicone muffin molds and freeze for 4 hours.

Remove fat bombs and enjoy!

Nutrition: Total Carbs: 1.3g Fiber: 0.2g Protein: 0.3g Fat: 7g

48   Crispy Coconut Bombs

Preparation time: 10 minutes

Cooking time: /

Freeze Time: 1-2 hours

Servings: 6

Ingredients:

14 ½ ounces coconut milk

¾ cup coconut oil

1 cup unsweetened coconut flakes

20 drops stevia

Directions:

Microwave your coconut oil for 20 seconds in microwave.

Mix in coconut milk and stevia in the hot oil.

Stir in coconut flakes and pour the mixture into molds.

Let it chill for 60 minutes in fridge.

Serve and enjoy!

Nutrition: Total Carbs: 2g Fiber: 0.5g Protein: 1g Fat: 13g

Calories: 123 Net Carbs: 1g

49   Pumpkin Pie Fat Bombs

Preparation time: 35 minutes

Cooking time: 5 minutes

Freeze Time: 3 hours

Servings: 12

Ingredients:

2 tablespoons coconut oil

1/3 cup pumpkin puree

1/3 cup almond oil

¼ cup almond oil

3 ounces sugar-free dark chocolate

1 ½ teaspoons pumpkin pie spice mix

Stevia to taste

Directions:

Melt almond oil and dark chocolate over a double boiler.

Take this mixture and layer the bottom of 12 muffin cups.

Freeze until the crust has set.

Meanwhile, take a saucepan and combine the rest of the ingredients.

Put the saucepan on low heat.

Heat until softened and mix well.

Pour this over the initial chocolate mixture.

Let it chill for at least 1 hour.

Nutrition:

Total Carbs: 3g Fiber: 1g Protein: 3g Fat: 13g Calories: 124

50 Sensational Lemonade Fat Bomb

Preparation time: 2 hours

Cooking time: Nil

Servings: 2

Ingredients:

½ lemon

4 ounces cream cheese

2 ounces almond butter

Salt to taste

2 teaspoons natural sweetener

Directions:

Take a fine grater and zest lemon.

Squeeze lemon juice into bowl with zest.

Add butter, cream cheese in a bowl and add zest, juice, salt, sweetener.

Mix well using a hand mixer until smooth.

Spoon mixture into molds and let them freeze for 2 hours.

Serve and enjoy!

Nutrition: Calories: 404 Fat: 43g Carbohydrates: 4g Protein: 4g

Conclusion

I hope this book will help motivate you to give the DASH diet a try if you haven't already. Regardless of which diet you try, I hope you will find the tips and tricks in this book helpful on your path to reach your health goals.

If you have other tricks and are aware of research that helps, please let me know. I am always updating my books to make sure they are as comprehensive as possible. We are all in this life together and it makes sense to help each other live it better.

CPSIA information can be obtained
at www.ICGtesting.com
Printed in the USA
BVHW070351230221
600781BV00007B/1396

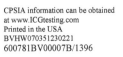